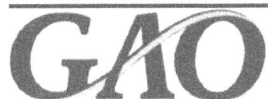

United States Government Accountability Office

Report to Congressional Committees

I0448128

November 2013

MINORITY AIDS INITIATIVE

Consolidation of Fragmented HIV/AIDS Funding Could Reduce Administrative Challenges

GAO Highlights

Highlights of GAO-14-84, a report to congressional committees

MINORITY AIDS INITIATIVE

Consolidation of Fragmented HIV/AIDS Funding Could Reduce Administrative Challenges

Why GAO Did This Study

According to CDC data, racial and ethnic minorities in the United States—particularly Blacks/African-Americans and Hispanics/Latinos—have been disproportionately affected by HIV/AIDS, representing 72 percent of new HIV infections and 74 percent of all AIDS diagnoses in 2011. In addition to core funding programs through CDC and HRSA that are intended to provide services to all qualifying individuals affected by HIV/AIDS, MAI seeks to improve HIV-related health outcomes and reduce health disparities for minority communities through the provision of grant funds. MAI grants are distributed to a variety of entities.

The Ryan White HIV/AIDS Treatment Extension Act of 2009 required GAO to (1) examine the services provided, population served, and administrative challenges faced by MAI grantees, and (2) describe the best practices identified by grantees and other stakeholders for community outreach and capacity building. GAO conducted a review of services reported in fiscal year 2011 MAI grantee annual reports from a generalizable sample of 100 grantees, and interviewed agency officials and other stakeholders. GAO also reviewed grant administrative requirements, and data on MAI grant amounts and populations served.

What GAO Recommends

To enhance HIV/AIDS services to minority populations, HHS should consolidate MAI funding into core HIV/AIDS funding and seek legislation as necessary to achieve a consolidated approach. HHS stated that GAO's recommendations align with the National HIV/AIDS Strategy.

View GAO-14-84. For more information, contact Marcia Crosse at (202) 512-7114 or crossem@gao.gov.

What GAO Found

Minority AIDS Initiative (MAI) grantees reported providing services similar to the medical services, support services, and HIV testing and prevention services provided with core HIV/AIDS funding, which is provided by the Health Resources and Services Administration (HRSA) and the Centers for Disease Control and Prevention (CDC) to grantees. In addition, MAI grantees faced administrative challenges managing HIV/AIDS funding that was fragmented across several grants. Various agencies within the Department of Health and Human Services (HHS) awarded MAI grants to grantees. The agencies included CDC, HRSA, the Substance Abuse and Mental Health Services Administration, and seven other offices within HHS. The MAI grantees in GAO's sample reported providing mostly support services with their MAI grants, similar to the types of support services grantees provided with core HIV/AIDS funding from CDC and HRSA. These support services included community outreach and education, and staff or provider training. Twenty percent of the grantees also reported providing medical services to their clients. According to the limited data HHS agencies and offices maintain on the demographics of the population served with MAI grants, the majority of recipients of MAI services were from racial and ethnic minority groups, as is also the case with recipients of services provided with core HIV/AIDS funds. MAI grantees faced administrative challenges because the fragmented nature of MAI and core HIV/AIDS funding required them to manage funding from several sources, each of which required them to complete multiple application and reporting requirements. For example, one city received nine HHS grants to provide HIV/AIDS services – six MAI grants and three core HIV/AIDS grants – and for each of these grants, that city had to complete separate administrative requirements. In this case, while HHS is funding all of the services, it is doing so across multiple funding streams, which raises the possibility of inefficiencies and requires unnecessarily duplicative application and reporting requirements of grantees that could otherwise be using their resources to provide needed services. Additionally, according to HRSA officials, these administrative challenges discouraged some grantees from applying for MAI grants. HRSA officials stated that some of the states receiving core HIV/AIDS grants chose not to request MAI grants because the grants' small size did not justify the additional reporting or other administrative requirements that would accompany them.

MAI grantee reports that GAO reviewed, as well as stakeholder organizations GAO interviewed, described a variety of best practices for community outreach and capacity building that at times led to improved client recruitment and improved capacity of community based organizations to serve communities disproportionately affected by HIV/AIDS. For instance, MAI grantees reported targeting specific communities, broadening outreach strategies, utilizing social media forums, and using various HIV testing strategies as best practices for community outreach that at times led to improved recruitment for HIV testing and other services. Grantees and some of the stakeholders reported that upgrading technology and providing training to grantee staff were the best methods to improve capacity to serve clients.

Contents

Letter		1
	Background	7
	Fragmented Funding for Similar Services to Similar Populations Resulted in Administrative Challenges for MAI Grantees	12
	MAI Grantees and Stakeholder Organizations Reported a Variety of Best Practices for Community Outreach and Capacity Building	20
	Conclusions	23
	Recommendations for Executive Action	23
	Agency Comments	24

Appendix I	Minority AIDS Initiative (MAI) Funding, Activities, and Grantees Funded, Fiscal Years 1999-2011	26

Appendix II	Methodology for Review of Minority AIDS Initiative (MAI) Services from Sample of MAI Annual Grantee Reports	37

Appendix III	Comments from the Department of Health and Human Services	41

Appendix IV	GAO Contact and Staff Acknowledgments	44

Tables

Table 1: Minority AIDS Initiative (MAI) Funding Allocations for Department of Health and Human Services (HHS) Agencies and Offices (in Millions of Dollars), Fiscal Year 2011	9
Table 2: The City of Chicago's MAI and Core HIV/AIDS Grant Administrative Requirements, Fiscal Year 2012	17
Table 3: Department of Health and Human Services (HHS) Minority AIDS Initiative (MAI) Funding (in Millions of Dollars), Fiscal Years 1999-2011	27
Table 4: Secretary's Minority AIDS Fund (SMAIF) Funding to HHS Offices (in Millions of Dollars), Fiscal Years 1999-2011	28

Table 5: Health Resources and Services Administration (HRSA) Minority AIDS Initiative Funding (in Millions of Dollars) and Number of Grantees, by Part, Fiscal Years 2007-2011   30

Table 6: Centers for Disease Control and Prevention (CDC) Minority AIDS Initiative (MAI) Funding (in Millions of Dollars) and Number of Grantees, Fiscal Years 2007-2011   31

Table 7: Substance Abuse and Mental Health Services Administration (SAMHSA) Minority AIDS Initiative (MAI) Funding (in Millions of Dollars) and Number of Grantees, Fiscal Years 2007-2011   33

Table 8: Indian Health Service (IHS) Secretary's Minority AIDS Initiative Funding (in Millions of Dollars) and Number of Grantees, Fiscal Years 2007-2011   33

Table 9: Office of HIV/AIDS and Infectious Disease Policy (OHAIDP) Secretary's Minority AIDS Initiative Funding (in Millions of Dollars) and Number of Grantees, Fiscal Years 2007-2011   34

Table 10: Office of Minority Health (OMH) Secretary's Minority AIDS Initiative Funding (in Millions of Dollars) and Number of Grantees, Fiscal Years 2007-2011   35

Table 11: Office of Population Affairs (OPA) Secretary's Minority AIDS Initiative Funding (in Millions of Dollars) and Number of Grantees, Fiscal Years 2007-2011   35

Table 12: Office on Women's Health (OWH) Secretary's Minority AIDS Initiative Funding (in Millions of Dollars) and Number of Grantees, Fiscal Years 2007-2011   36

Table 13: Regional Health Administrators (RHA) Secretary's Minority AIDS Initiative Funding (in Millions of Dollars) and Number of Grantees, Fiscal Years 2007-2011   36

Table 14: Categories of Services and Best Practices Identified in MAI Annual Grantee Reports   38

Abbreviations

AIDS	acquired immunodeficiency syndrome
CARE Act	Ryan White Comprehensive AIDS Resources Emergency Act of 1990
CBO	community-based organization
CDC	Centers for Disease Control and Prevention
HHS	Department of Health and Human Services
HIV	human immunodeficiency virus
HRSA	Health Resources and Services Administration
IHS	Indian Health Service
MAI	Minority AIDS Initiative
OAH	Office of Adolescent Health
OHAIDP	HHS Office of HIV/AIDS and Infectious Disease Policy
OMH	Office of Minority Health
OPA	Office of Population Affairs
OWH	Office on Women's Health
RHA	Regional Health Administrators
SAMHSA	Substance Abuse and Mental Health Services Administration
SMAIF	Secretary's Minority AIDS Initiative Fund

November 22, 2013

The Honorable Tom Harkin
Chairman
The Honorable Lamar Alexander
Ranking Member
Committee on Health, Education, Labor and Pensions
United States Senate

The Honorable Fred Upton
Chairman
The Honorable Henry Waxman
Ranking Member
Committee on Energy and Commerce
House of Representatives

An estimated 1.2 million people in the United States were living with human immunodeficiency virus (HIV) infections in 2012, and approximately 50,000 new infections occur annually. Since the first cases of acquired immunodeficiency syndrome (AIDS) were reported in June 1981, more than 600,000 people with AIDS have died. Racial and ethnic minorities in the United States —particularly African-Americans and Hispanics/Latinos—have been disproportionately affected by HIV/AIDS.[1] According to the most recent data from the Centers for Disease Control and Prevention (CDC), part of the Department of Health and Human Services (HHS), racial and ethnic minorities represented 72 percent of new HIV infections and 74 percent of all AIDS diagnoses in 2011.[2]

Two agencies within HHS, the Health Resources and Services Administration (HRSA) and CDC, administer grant programs that provide

---

[1] HIV is the virus that causes AIDS. We use the common term HIV/AIDS to refer to HIV disease, inclusive of cases that have progressed to AIDS. When we use these terms alone, HIV refers to the disease without the presence of AIDS, and AIDS refers exclusively to HIV disease that has progressed to AIDS.

[2] CDC releases data on the number of diagnoses of HIV infection annually and the total number AIDS cases annually in its surveillance reports. Data from 2011 are the most recent available for these measures.

core HIV/AIDS funding for HIV/AIDS services.[3] HRSA awards core HIV/AIDS grants pursuant to the Ryan White Comprehensive AIDS Resources Emergency Act of 1990 (CARE Act), which was enacted to address the treatment needs of uninsured and underinsured persons living with HIV/AIDS.[4] In fiscal year 2011, HRSA's budget for core CARE Act programs for HIV/AIDS treatment through the provision of medical services, support services, and education was approximately $2.1 billion.

Independent of HRSA's core grant programs under the CARE Act, CDC's Division of HIV/AIDS Policy awards core HIV/AIDS grants for prevention programs, research and evaluation, surveillance, and policy development to reduce the impact of HIV/AIDS. In fiscal year 2011, CDC's budget for its core HIV/AIDS programs was approximately $666.4 million. Goals for CDC's core HIV/AIDS funding in fiscal year 2011 included decreasing annual HIV incidence, decreasing the HIV transmission rate, increasing the proportion of HIV-infected people in the United States who know they are infected, improving HIV/AIDS surveillance, and ensuring that all persons diagnosed with HIV are linked to care.

In addition to the core HIV/AIDS grant programs, CDC, HRSA, and numerous other HHS agencies and offices award grants to implement the Minority AIDS Initiative (MAI). First known as the Congressional Black Caucus Initiative, MAI originated in 1998 in response to provisions in a house conference report accompanying the Omnibus Consolidated and Emergency Supplemental Appropriations Act, 1999.[5] The conference report instructed HRSA to target funds to reduce HIV-related treatment outcome disparities in communities of color, noting that this funding

---

[3]We use the term "core funding" to refer to those funding programs administered by CDC and HRSA that are intended to provide services to all qualifying individuals affected by HIV/AIDS, as opposed to targeted funding programs within HHS's Minority Aids Initiative.

[4]Pub. L. No. 101-381, 104 Stat. 576 (codified, as amended, at 42 U.S.C. §§ 300ff through 300ff-121). The 1990 CARE Act added title XXVI to the Public Health Service Act. Unless otherwise indicated, references to the CARE Act refer to current title XXVI. The CARE Act programs have been reauthorized by the Ryan White CARE Act Amendments of 1996 (Pub. L. No. 104-146, 110 Stat. 1346), the Ryan White CARE Act Amendments of 2000 (Pub. L. No. 106-345, 114 Stat. 1319), the Ryan White HIV/AIDS Treatment Modernization Act of 2006 (Pub. L. No. 109-415, 120 Stat. 2767), and the Ryan White HIV/AIDS Treatment Extension Act of 2009 (Pub. L. No. 111-87, 123 Stat. 2885).

[5]Pub. L. No. 105-277, 112 Stat. 2681 (1998).

should be used to complement existing and previously planned targeted HIV/AIDS minority activities.[6]

In the context of HIV/AIDS grants, applicants may be eligible to receive core HIV/AIDS grants and/or MAI grants. These grant programs carry different administrative requirements that grantees must observe for each of the separate grants they may receive. Agencies and offices that administer grants maintain these requirements to ensure that the funds are being used in the way intended by the grant program.

The Ryan White HIV/AIDS Treatment Extension Act of 2009 required us to report on MAI and related issues.[7] In this report, we (1) examine the services provided, population served, and administrative challenges faced by MAI grantees, and (2) describe the best practices identified by grantees and other stakeholders for community outreach and capacity building of CBOs serving the communities that are disproportionately affected by HIV/AIDS. The Ryan White HIV/AIDS Treatment Extension Act of 2009 also requires us to report on the history of MAI activities within each relevant HHS agency and office to provide a description of activities conducted and types of grantees funded. We provide information from prior years on MAI funding, activities, and grantees in appendix I.

To examine the services provided, population served, and administrative challenges faced by MAI grantees, we interviewed all ten HHS agencies and offices that awarded MAI grants in fiscal year 2011. These HHS agencies and offices include HRSA, the primary federal agency for improving access to health care services for uninsured, isolated or medically vulnerable individuals; the Substance Abuse and Mental Health Services Administration (SAMHSA), which leads public health efforts to advance the behavioral health of the nation; CDC, which seeks to protect health and promote quality of life through the prevention and control of disease, injury, and disability; the Indian Health Service (IHS), which provides federal health services to American Indians and Alaska Natives; the Office of Population Affairs (OPA), which aims to be the leader in family planning and reproductive health care services, training and research; the Office of Minority Health (OMH); which aims to improve the

---

[6]H.R. Conf. Rep. No. 105-825, at 1265 (1998).

[7]Pub. L. No. 111-87, § 2(g), 123 Stat. 2885, 2887 (codified at 42 U.S.C. § 300ff-86).

health of racial and ethnic minority populations through the development of health policies and programs; the Office of HIV/AIDS and Infectious Disease Policy (OHAIDP), which advises HHS officials on the implementation and development of policies, programs, and activities related to HIV/AIDS and other infectious diseases; the Office on Women's Health (OWH), which seeks to improve the health and sense of well-being of women and girls; the Regional Health Administrators (RHA), which seeks to perform essential functions for HHS in prevention, preparedness, and agency-wide coordination; and the Office of Adolescent Health (OAH), which seeks to improve the health and well being of adolescents. We also interviewed staff from six stakeholder organizations, including national HIV/AIDS organizations that represent MAI grantees: the Black AIDS Institute, Latino Commission on AIDS, National Alliance of State and Territorial AIDS Directors, National Council of Urban Indian Health, National Minority AIDS Council, and National Native American AIDS Prevention Center. In addition, we interviewed the Kaiser Family Foundation, a subject matter expert. We interviewed these organizations to obtain their perspectives on MAI. Information we obtained from these interviews is not generalizable. We conducted a review of MAI services reported in MAI annual grantee reports from a generalizable sample of 100 MAI grantees from fiscal year 2011.[8] To select our sample, we created a list of all MAI grantees from the ten HHS agencies and offices that awarded MAI grants in fiscal year 2011 and then selected a generalizable sample of 100 grantees from these agencies and offices.[9] We then obtained MAI annual grantee reports for these grantees from the respective agencies and offices and used NVivo software to identify the types of MAI services in these reports (app. II

---

[8]We obtained fiscal year 2011 MAI annual grantee reports because this was the most recent information available for most agencies and offices. Some grantees had not yet submitted their fiscal year 2011 reports at the time we did our work. Where this was the case, we used the fiscal year 2010 reports. MAI grantees submit annual grantee reports to the agency that awarded their MAI grants that typically include information on the types of services they provided with their MAI funds. Grantees that receive more than one MAI grant often have to submit a separate report to each agency from which they receive grants.

[9]We identified a total of 1067 organizations awarded MAI grants by the ten HHS agencies and offices in fiscal year 2011. In addition to grants, some agencies may have awarded MAI funding to recipients through other mechanisms such as cooperative agreements, contracts, or interagency agreements. We have treated these recipients as "grantees" for purposes of this report regardless of the funding mechanism by which they received their funds.

provides more detail on our sample design.).[10] Estimates of the services provided and population served from this sample are generalizable to the population of MAI grantees. We summarize the statistical precision of our estimates using a 95 percent confidence interval, which is the interval that would contain the population value in 95 percent of the samples we could have drawn. Since the size of the confidence intervals varies widely across the estimates, we specify these intervals where we refer to the estimates. We categorized MAI services described in the grantee reports into six categories. We then analyzed and compared the services identified in these categories by HHS agency and office, grant amount, source of grant, and organizational type. We also reviewed agency guidance on which services grantees are expected to provide with their MAI and core HIV/AIDS grants.

In addition, to identify the population served by MAI, we obtained and reviewed the available demographic data on the race and ethnicity of the clients served with MAI grants as well as aggregate historical funding data that we requested and obtained from HHS agencies and offices for fiscal years 2007-2012. Some agencies and offices could not provide demographic data on their clients, but we assessed the reliability of the demographic data that the agencies and offices could provide by interviewing agency officials about how their demographic data was collected, and we also discussed any inconsistencies we found in the data. We found the data provided to be sufficiently reliable for presenting information about the race and ethnicity of MAI grantee populations. We also obtained, reviewed, and analyzed the core HIV/AIDS grant amounts that MAI grantees in our sample were awarded in order to understand the total amount of HIV/AIDS funding that MAI grantees received. We then compared the core HIV/AIDS grant amounts to their MAI grant amounts. To determine core HIV/AIDS grant amounts, we used CDC and HRSA funding data in addition to publicly available funding data. We compared publically available data to data provided to us, and confirmed the data with the agencies where there were discrepancies. We found these data to be reliable for our purposes.

Furthermore, to assist us in reviewing the administrative challenges faced by MAI grantees, we evaluated grantee administrative requirements

---

[10]NVivo is a qualitative data analysis software system that allows organization and analysis of information from a variety of sources including complex nonnumeric or unstructured data.

including applications and reporting requirements for MAI and core HIV/AIDS grants, and considered our past work on federal programs or activities government-wide that have evidence of fragmentation, overlap, or duplication.[11] In that work, we found that the presence of fragmentation can lead to instances of overlap and duplication among government agencies or programs that have similar goals or activities.

To describe the best practices identified by grantees for community outreach and capacity building of CBOs serving communities disproportionately affected by HIV/AIDS, we conducted a review of MAI annual grantee reports from our generalizable sample of 100 MAI grantees using NVivo software in order to identify and categorize what grantees considered to be best practices. Specifically, we identified and analyzed MAI services that grantees considered were best practices, which included best practices for community outreach or capacity building of CBOs that serve communities disproportionally affected by HIV/AIDS. We defined the term best practices to include any successes, lessons learned, or challenges overcome by grantees regarding their MAI activities. Because grantees generally were not required to discuss best practices in their MAI annual grantee reports, we cannot estimate the proportion of grantees identifying such practices. Instead, we can simply count the number of best practices reported in our sample that we identified using our definition of best practices. As a result, our estimates are not generalizable for this purpose, unlike our estimates of services provided. In addition, we also obtained information on best practices for community outreach and capacity building from the six stakeholder organizations and one subject matter expert we interviewed.

We conducted this performance audit from October 2012 to November 2013 in accordance with generally accepted government auditing standards. Those standards require that we plan and perform the audit to obtain sufficient, appropriate evidence to provide a reasonable basis for our findings and conclusions based on our audit objectives. We believe

---

[11]Fragmentation occurs when one or more federal agencies or agency organizations are involved in the same broad area of national need and opportunities exist to improve service delivery. Overlap occurs when multiple agencies or programs have similar goals, engage in similar activities or strategies to achieve them, or target similar beneficiaries. Duplication occurs when two or more agencies or programs are engaged in the same activities or provide the same services to the same beneficiaries. See GAO, *2013 Annual Report: Actions Needed to Reduce Fragmentation, Overlap, and Duplication and Achieve Other Financial Benefits*, GAO-13-279SP (Washington, D.C.: Apr. 9, 2013).

that the evidence obtained provides a reasonable basis for our findings and conclusions based on our audit objectives.

Background

History of MAI

MAI was established in 1998 in response to growing concern about the impact of HIV/AIDS on racial and ethnic minorities in the United States. According to the most recent CDC data, there were an estimated 23,734 AIDS diagnoses in 2011 among persons of minority races/ethnicities, accounting for 74 percent of total AIDS diagnoses in the United States and dependent areas; these data reflect an overall trend present since 1994. National HIV/AIDS data indicate that since 1994 minorities have become a significant majority of persons with HIV/AIDS. In 2011, Blacks/African-Americans accounted for 13 percent of the U.S. population, but accounted for 49 percent of AIDS diagnoses; Hispanics/Latinos accounted for 17 percent of the population, but accounted for 21 percent of AIDS diagnoses; and Caucasians/Whites accounted for 74 percent of the population, but accounted for 26 percent of AIDS diagnoses.[12]

HRSA's MAI program was codified into law as part of the 2006 reauthorization of the CARE Act.[13] To be eligible for MAI grants under the CARE Act, grantees must also have received CARE Act grants under Parts A through D or F, these MAI grants provide funding in addition to

---

[12]Those who identify as Hispanic or Latino may be any race, therefore CDC data on AIDS diagnoses may combine Hispanics/Latinos with other races. "Hispanic or Latino," as defined in the 2010 Census, refers to a person of Cuban, Mexican, Puerto Rican, South or Central American, or other Spanish culture or origin regardless of race. Additionally, Asian-Americans accounted for two percent of the AIDS diagnoses, and Native American/Alaskan Native/Native Hawaiian/other Pacific Islanders accounted for less than two percent of the AIDS diagnoses in 2011.

[13]Pub. L. No. 109-415, § 603, 120 Stat. 2767, 2818 (codified at 300ff-121).

core HIV/AIDs grants awarded by HRSA under other provisions of the CARE Act.[14]

Other HHS agencies and offices, including HRSA, continue to carry out MAI grant programs separate from the statutory MAI program that HRSA implements under the CARE Act. In particular, CDC, SAMHSA, and the Office of the Secretary also award MAI grants to provide services for communities disproportionally affected by HIV/AIDS. CDC and SAMHSA award MAI grants directly to grantees. In contrast, MAI funds administered by the Office of the Secretary, referred to as the Secretary's MAI Fund (SMAIF), are distributed by the Office of HIV/AIDS and Infectious Disease Policy (OHAIDP) to HRSA, CDC, SAMHSA, and seven other HHS agencies and offices. These agencies and offices, in turn, award SMAIF grants. MAI and SMAIF funding are often provided to the same grantees that receive core HIV/AIDS funding.

MAI Funding Allocations in Fiscal Year 2011

Three HHS agencies, HRSA, SAMSHA, and CDC, allocate a portion of their respective annual appropriations to carry out MAI programs. In fiscal year 2011, CDC, HRSA, and SAMHSA allocated approximately $363.7 million of their respective appropriations for MAI programs. CDC, HRSA, and SAMHSA use this funding to award grants for the provision of services to racial and ethnic minorities with HIV/AIDS.[15] In addition, the Office of the Secretary receives an annual line item MAI appropriation, which it calls SMAIF. The Office of the Secretary received a $52.8 million appropriation for SMAIF funding in fiscal year 2011. OHAIDP distributed this funding on behalf of the Office of the Secretary to ten HHS agencies and offices within HHS, including HRSA, CDC, and SAMHSA, for a

---

[14]HRSA awards core HIV/AIDS grants under Parts A through D and Part F of the CARE Act. Part A provides for grants to selected metropolitan areas that have been disproportionately affected by the HIV/AIDS epidemic. Part B provides for grants to states and territories to improve the quality, availability, and organization of HIV/AIDS services. Part C provides for grants to public and private nonprofit entities to provide early intervention services such as HIV testing and ambulatory care. Part D provides for grants to programs for family-centered comprehensive care to children, youth, and women and their families. Part F provides for grants for demonstration and evaluation of innovative models of HIV/AIDS care delivery for hard-to-reach populations and training of health care providers. In addition to the core HIV/AIDs grants provided under Part F of the CARE Act, Part F also contains the provisions that form the statutory basis for supplemental MAI grants under the CARE Act, which are codified at 42 U.S.C.§ 300ff-121.

[15]CDC may also provide funds to grantees through cooperative agreements and contracts. We include these funds in our counts of grants.

variety of activities to address HIV/AIDS in racial and ethnic minority communities. In turn, these agencies and offices awarded SMAIF grants and cooperative agreements to the same types of organizations and entities that receive other MAI funding to provide services. HRSA's SMAIF funding is in addition to the amounts it receives in order to make MAI grants under the CARE Act. (See table 1 for fiscal year 2011 MAI funding.)

Table 1: Minority AIDS Initiative (MAI) Funding Allocations for Department of Health and Human Services (HHS) Agencies and Offices (in Millions of Dollars), Fiscal Year 2011

HHS Agency or Office	Agency MAI Allocations[a]	HHS Allocation of MAI (SMAIF) Appropriation[b]
Health Resources and Services Administration (HRSA)	$153.4	$7.7
Substance Abuse and Mental Health Services Administration (SAMHSA)	$116.7	$5.9
Centers for Disease Control and Prevention (CDC)	$93.6	$10.4
Indian Health Service (IHS)		$4.2
Office of Population Affairs (OPA)		$7.2
Office of Minority Health (OMH)		$5.5
Office of HIV/AIDS and Infectious Disease Policy (OHAIDP)		$3.4
Office on Women's Health (OWH)		$3.4
Regional Health Administrators (RHA)		$2.0
Office of Adolescent Health (OAH)		$0.2
Total	**$363.7**	**$52.8[c]**

Source: GAO analysis of HHS data.

Note: Dollar amounts are rounded to one decimal point.

[a]HRSA, SAMHSA, and CDC allocate MAI funds from their respective annual appropriations.

[b]The HHS Office of the Secretary receives an annual MAI appropriation which is referred to as the Secretary's Minority AIDS Fund (SMAIF), that it distributes to ten HHS agencies, which include HRSA, SAMHSA, and CDC.

[c]According to agency officials, the expenses associated with the administration of SMAIF funding were $2.9M in fiscal year 2011 which we include in the HHS Allocation of MAI (SMAIF) Appropriation.

MAI grantees include a wide variety of organizations.[16] MAI grantees include health departments, state and local governments, tribal governments, community health centers, hospitals and medical centers, CBOs, colleges and universities, AIDS Education and Training Centers, and national HIV/AIDS organizations such as the National Minority AIDS Council.[17] MAI grantees also include commercial vendors and businesses that are awarded contracts to conduct evaluations of MAI programs. Some MAI grantees also receive core HIV/AIDS funding. Where this is the case, MAI grants generally account for a small percentage of the grantee's funding to provide HIV/AIDS services.

Core HIV/AIDS and MAI Budget Request and Allocation Process

As part of the federal budget process, HHS requests core HIV/AIDS funding and MAI funding, which Congress provides under different appropriations provisions. After its annual budget is enacted, HHS exercises discretion in allocating core HIV/AIDS funding and MAI funding to the extent authorized by law.

With respect to the CARE Act, annual appropriations acts provide an amount for all CARE Act programs, as well as requirements to make certain sums available for implementing specific parts of the CARE Act such as Parts A and B.[18] Annual CARE Act appropriations have not directed specific amounts for the MAI program, although the authorizing legislation provides a schedule of amounts to be reserved for supplemental MAI grants from any amounts appropriated for the MAI program.[19] HRSA derives its annual MAI budget allocation based on the schedule of amounts provided in the authorizing legislation.

Congress has not enacted specific appropriations provisions applicable to core HIV/AIDS programs administered by CDC or the separate MAI programs administered by CDC and SAMSHA. As a result, these

---

[16]When we use the term MAI grantees, we are referring to all grantees that receive MAI funding, including those that receive SMAIF funding.

[17]Sixteen AIDS Education and Training Centers provide HIV/AIDS education to health professionals such as nurses and physicians. The AIDS Education and Training Centers are authorized by the CARE Act.

[18]For example, see Department of Health and Human Services Appropriations Act, 2010, Pub. L. No. 111-117, div. D, title II, 123 Stat. 3034, 3239-3240 (2009).

[19]42 U.S.C. § 300ff-121(b).

agencies exercise discretion in making allocation decisions for their respective programs, which may be influenced by any applicable committee report language accompanying their annual appropriations acts.

During the budget request process, HHS also requests general departmental management funds for the Office of the Secretary, including an amount for prevention and treatment activities known as SMAIF. Congress has provided an annual line item appropriation to the Office of the Secretary for this purpose, without specifying how HHS is to allocate these funds. As a result, HHS exercises discretion in allocating this funding to numerous agencies and offices to implement separate MAI grant programs.

MAI Administrative Requirements

About three-quarters of MAI grantees submit applications, and about a quarter are not required to submit an application. The application process generally consists of an application or request for funding that includes a written description of the services the grantee plans to provide using the MAI grant. For example, SAMHSA grantees are required to submit applications which provide details on how grantees plan to spend their MAI grants on programs related to substance abuse and mental health services. Agencies and offices that award MAI grants evaluate whether to fund grantees based upon whether or not their planned services are consistent with MAI. However, grant amounts may be determined by a formula that considers the number of racial and ethnic minorities reported to have HIV that live in the area the grantee serves. About a quarter of MAI grantees receive core HIV/AIDS funding and are not required to submit any application for MAI grants. In these instances, the amount of the MAI grant is also based upon a formula that considers the number of racial and ethnic minorities reported to have HIV that live in areas served by the grantee.

According to HHS officials, MAI grantees are required to report to their funding agency on how they use their MAI grants. These reports generally include a description of the services they provided with the grants and an accounting of the grants themselves. HHS officials stated that MAI grantees are generally required to submit reports at least annually, but some are required to submit reports more frequently. HHS officials stated that some grantees report on their use of MAI grants as part of their reporting on their use of core HIV/AIDS grants. HHS agencies use these reports to evaluate whether the services grantees provided to racial and ethnic minorities with HIV/AIDS met the objectives they outlined in their applications.

Fragmented Funding for Similar Services to Similar Populations Resulted in Administrative Challenges for MAI Grantees

MAI grantees reported providing services similar to those provided with core HIV/AIDS grants. MAI and core HIV/AIDS grantees provided services primarily to minorities. MAI grants were often part of fragmented HIV/AIDS funding streams that carried separate administrative requirements that caused administrative challenges for MAI grantees.

MAI Grantees Provided Services Similar to Those Provided with Core HIV/AIDS Funding

MAI grantees in our sample reported providing mostly support services, similar to the types of support services grantees provided with core HIV/AIDS grants. These support services included community outreach and education, and staff or provider training.[20] A fraction of the grantees reported providing medical services to their clients.

Based on our review of the annual reports submitted by 100 MAI grantees in our sample, we found

- Eighty-one percent of grantees reported providing community outreach and education services for the purposes of recruiting and retaining clients to HIV/AIDS services.[21] For example, grantees reported using social media platforms, including Facebook and Twitter, to recruit and retain individuals into care and holding community HIV/AIDS awareness events.

- Seventy-two percent of grantees reported providing assistance to clients including care coordination, case management, or referrals to care.[22] Activities also included assisting clients with social services such as housing, employment, and post-HIV test counseling.

---

[20]Grantees reported they either provided these services to clients directly or helped providers to deliver MAI services.

[21]The 95 percent confidence interval of this estimate ranges from 72 to 89 percent.

[22]The 95 percent confidence interval of this estimate ranges from 63 to 81 percent.

- Sixty-nine percent of grantees reported providing clients with HIV/AIDS or other related illnesses testing services, such as rapid HIV testing.[23]

- Fifty-eight percent of grantees reported providing or receiving training for grantee staff, providers, or other organizations affiliated with the grantee, such as training to keep providers informed about HIV related clinical service guidelines.[24]

- Twenty percent of grantees reported using MAI grants to provide core medical services to clients.[25] For example, grantees provided primary and outpatient medical care to HIV/AIDS-infected clients and substance abuse treatment or counseling to clients.[26] Two stakeholders we interviewed believed MAI funds have not been targeted to medical services, and are generally too small to support providing medical services.

The services provided by MAI grantees were similar to those provided by grantees awarded HRSA's and CDC's core HIV/AIDS funding. HRSA's fiscal year 2011 budget justification to Congress indicated that core HIV/AIDS funds were used to provide clients with medical care such as primary health care; assisting clients by providing early intervention services; family support services; training for health care providers; and other support services. CDC described using its core HIV/AIDS funding to provide support services that included training clients by enhancing prevention services among the most affected communities. The services described included assisting clients by integrating and providing linkage to care services and expanding HIV testing. CDC also described community outreach and education services that included developing social marketing campaigns.

The services that MAI grantees reported providing are consistent with available guidance. Guidance for MAI grantees varied considerably across the agencies and offices that receive MAI funding. However, agency guidance generally instructed grantees to provide services similar

---

[23]The 95 percent confidence interval of this estimate ranges from 61 to 76 percent.

[24]The 95 percent confidence interval of this estimate ranges from 51 to 66 percent.

[25]The 95 percent confidence interval of this estimate ranges from 13 to 30 percent.

[26]The maximum 95 percent confidence interval of these estimates is 15 percent.

to those provided with core HIV/AIDS grants and instructed grantees to ensure that they provided services within racial and ethnic minority communities. Some agencies and offices that award MAI grants provide specific guidance to grantees on how to use those grants, while others provide guidance in the form of application and reporting instructions.

Available Data Suggest MAI and Core HIV/AIDS Grantees Provide Services Primarily to Minorities

The limited demographic information available from the HHS agencies and offices that could provide data suggests that the majority of those served with both MAI and core HIV/AIDS grants are racial and ethnic minorities.[27] This is consistent with the current distribution of HIV/AIDS in the United States. HHS officials also said that the majority of clients served by MAI grantees are minorities. However, the demographic data are not consistently tracked. Agency officials said that HHS did not require them to request and compile demographic data from MAI or core HIV/AIDS grantees in fiscal year 2011. HHS agencies and offices were only able to provide us data for 54 percent of MAI grantees in fiscal year 2011, representing 34 percent of all MAI funding. These data suggest that HHS's assessment is likely correct. SAMHSA data indicated that 70 percent of its MAI service recipients were minorities in fiscal year 2011. Available demographic data from three offices that receive SMAIF funding— OPA, OMH, and OWH—indicated that over 80 percent of their MAI service recipients were minorities. IHS data indicated it served a MAI population that was 100 percent American Indian/Alaska Native.

HRSA is the only agency that could provide demographic data on the recipients of services funded by core HIV/AIDS grants but these data combined recipients of services funded by core HIV/AIDS grants with recipients of services funded by MAI grants. Although the data included recipients of services from MAI grants, they provide a good indication of the demographics of recipients of services from core HIV/AIDS grants because MAI grants only amount to 7 percent of core HIV/AIDS funding.[28] The data provided by HRSA, which accounted for 76 percent of core

---

[27]Those who identify as Hispanic or Latino may be any race, therefore agency data may combine Hispanics with other races when determining the number and percent of minorities served. "Hispanic or Latino," as defined in the 2010 Census, refers to a person of Cuban, Mexican, Puerto Rican, South or Central American, or other Spanish culture or origin regardless of race.

[28]CDC could not provide demographic data on the recipients of services funded by core HIV/AIDS funds.

HIV/AIDS grants across HHS agencies and offices, indicate that 73 percent of the recipients were minority. Specifically, 47 percent were African-Americans/Blacks, 22 percent identified as Hispanics, and 4 percent identified as either Asian, American Indian/Alaska Native, Native Hawaiian/Pacific Islander or Multi-racial.[29] This is consistent with the overall demographics of the HIV-positive population in the United States, in which racial and ethnic minorities represented 72 percent of new HIV infections and 74 percent of all AIDS diagnoses in 2011.While the data are insufficient to conclusively determine the extent to which each program serves minority clients, the data suggest that both primarily serve minority populations.

MAI Grantees Face Challenges Resulting from the Administrative Requirements of Fragmented Funding Streams

MAI and core HIV/AIDS funding is often fragmented across several grants, sometimes from several different HHS offices or agencies. In past work, we have concluded that funding is fragmented when more than one agency or more than one organization within an agency provides funding in the same broad areas of national need, and opportunities exist to improve service delivery. In this work, we identified approaches that agencies can take to improve efficiency. These approaches include streamlining or consolidating management or operational processes to make them more cost-effective.[30] MAI and core HIV/AIDS funding is fragmented because numerous agencies and offices in HHS receive it and all provide services to respond to the same area of national need. The National HIV/AIDS Strategy of 2010 noted this issue as one that could complicate the coordination of HIV/AIDS programs. The Strategy stated that "HIV service providers often receive funding from multiple sources with different grant application processes and funding schedules, and varied reporting requirements."[31] As noted earlier, Congress has not enacted specific appropriations provisions applicable to core HIV/AIDS programs administered by CDC or the separate MAI programs administered by CDC and SAMHSA. As a result, these agencies exercise discretion in making allocation decisions for their respective core HIV/AIDS and MAI programs, which may be influenced by applicable

---

[29]These data are based on CARE Act Parts A, B, C, and D data.

[30]GAO, *2013 Annual Report: Actions Needed to Reduce Fragmentation, Overlap, and Duplication and Achieve Other Financial Benefits*, GAO-13-279SP (Washington, D.C.: Apr. 9, 2013), 3.

[31]The White House, *National HIV/AIDS Strategy for the United States* (July 2010), 42.

committee report language accompanying their annual appropriations acts. Additionally, annual line item appropriations for SMAIF programs do not specify how HHS is to allocate these funds to implement MAI. Thus, HHS can exercise discretion to consolidate disparate MAI funding streams. In addition, HHS could seek legislation to amend the CARE Act or other law, as necessary, to enable HHS to further consolidate amounts directed at MAI programs into core HIV/AIDs programs.

The fragmented nature of MAI and core HIV/AIDS funding caused administrative challenges for grantees by often forcing grantees to manage grants from several sources. These funding sources required them to complete multiple administrative requirements. The duplication and fragmentation of these requirements across the grant sources create inefficiencies for the grantee that could be providing needed HIV/AIDS services instead of using resources to complete multiple administrative requirements. In fiscal year 2011, 56 percent, or 596, of the 1067 MAI grantees received several HIV/AIDS grants, including at least one MAI grant and one core HIV/AIDS grant. Of these 596 MAI grantees, 167 received a core HIV/AIDS grant from both CDC and HRSA.

For example, the city of Chicago received nine grants from HHS to provide HIV/AIDS services. These include six MAI grants—one grant from MAI Part A and one grant from MAI Part C, and four MAI grants from CDC and SAMHSA, one from each agency's MAI allocation and one from each agency's SMAIF funding. In addition, Chicago received three core HIV/AIDS grants—one from CARE Act Part A, one from CARE Act Part C, and one from CDC. Chicago is required to submit a report or application for one of its HIV/AIDS grants in most months of the year and in some months, they are required to produce multiple submissions. While the specific services Chicago provided with the 9 grants varied, all of the grants were used to provide HIV/AIDS treatment or prevention services to residents of the city of Chicago. (See table 2.) Other cities with a similar array of grants include Philadelphia, San Francisco, Los Angeles, and New York City. MAI grantees face challenges in managing the multiple administrative requirements for each of these grants.

Table 2: The City of Chicago's MAI and Core HIV/AIDS Grant Administrative Requirements, Fiscal Year 2012

Administrative Requirement	Due Date, Fiscal Year 2012	Source of Grant Type of Grant
Targeted Capacity Expansion Grant Application	June 13, 2011[a]	SAMHSA
The grant application is required for the 12 Metropolitan Statistical Areas and Metropolitan Divisions most impacted by HIV/AIDS. Award amounts vary based on the size of the population most at risk for or living with HIV in the jurisdiction, but grantees are required to submit documentation of intent to provide required services, ability to collect data and measure performance, and budget information.		MAI
Minority AIDS Initiative Annual Plan	October 17, 2011	HRSA
The primary purpose of the Part A MAI Annual Plan is to ensure grants are used to link minority clients to HIV care services. The plan is to include a planned timeframe for delivering services; a description of service goals and objectives; the racial and ethnic communities to be served, and the number of service units to be provided during the reporting period.		MAI, Part A
CARE Act Part A Grant Application	November 1, 2011	HRSA
The CARE Act application is required for all 52 CARE Act Part A grantees. The application requires grantees to report information on current and new program initiatives. The application also outlines the reporting requirements and other documentation required from grantees.		Core HIV/AIDS funding, CARE Act Part A
Maintenance of Effort Expenditures Report	December 5, 2011	HRSA
The maintenance of effort expenditures report is used to ensure grantees have maintained level expenditures for two consecutive grant years. The expenditures must be based on the local budget items.		Core HIV/AIDS funding, CARE Act Part A
Program Terms Report	December 5, 2011	HRSA
The program terms report includes a planned allocation report, budget and budget justification narrative, an implementation plan, the Consolidated List of Contractors, and the Contract Review Certification.[b]		Core HIV/AIDS funding, CARE Act Part A
Unobligated Balance Estimate and Carryover Request	January 1, 2012	HRSA
The CARE Act provides that base and supplemental grant funds were available for obligation by the grantee for a 1-year period beginning on the first day of the grant year. It also requires HRSA to cancel any unobligated balances not subject to a waiver at the end of the grant year, recover funds that had been disbursed to grantees, and redistribute these funds to grantees in need as supplemental grants. Grantees must estimate their unobligated balances during the grant year and provide final amounts in their federal financial report. Grantees may request to carryover funds for one additional grant year.		Core HIV/AIDS funding, CARE Act Part A
CARE Act HIV/AIDS Program Services Report	March 15, 2012	HRSA
The CARE Act HIV/AIDS program services report provides information on services provided by grantees and service providers to HRSA. Additionally, grantees and service providers use this report to provide information on clients, including their demographic status, services received and HIV clinical information.		Core HIV/AIDS funding, CARE Act Part A

Administrative Requirement	Due Date, Fiscal Year 2012	Source of Grant Type of Grant
CARE Act Part A Comprehensive Plan	May 21, 2012	HRSA
The comprehensive plan is a requirement that is due every 3 years at the beginning of the grant year. The plan is to be used as a "road map" for the maintenance and improvement of the grantee's system of care. Grantees are required to include appropriate strategies, goals, and timelines.		Core HIV/AIDS funding, CARE Act Part A
Final Expenditure Table, including MAI Expenditures	June 28, 2012	HRSA
This expenditure table serves as a monitoring tool to identify the use of grants at the end of the grant period. It identifies service categories that have been delivered, the use of carry-over grants, and identifies trends in the amount of CARE Act grants being used to deliver these services.		Core HIV/AIDS funding, CARE Act Part A
Annual Progress Report	June 28, 2012[c]	HRSA
The Annual Progress Report is to inform HRSA of the progress made in the administration of Ryan White programs; to identify accomplishments and challenges in meeting established goals and objectives; and to address grantees' need for technical assistance.		Core HIV/AIDS funding, CARE Act Part A
Report on Expenditures for Women, Infants, Children and Youth	July 28, 2012	HRSA
The report on expenditures for Women, Infants, Children and Youth is a requirement used to determine that a grantee allocates resources for women, infants, children, and youth at no less than the percentage constituted by the ratio of the population of women, infants, children, and youth with HIV/AIDS to the general populations with HIV/AIDS.		Core HIV/AIDS funding, CARE Act Part A
Federal Financial Report	July 30, 2012	HRSA
The Federal Financial Report outlines the grantee's outlays, unliquidated obligations, total federal share, and final unobligated balance.		Core HIV/AIDS funding, CARE Act Part A
Minority AIDS Initiative Annual Report	January 31, 2013	HRSA
CARE Act Part A grantees receiving MAI funds must submit two components of the MAI Report annually: (1) the MAI Annual Plan for the use of these funds, and (2) the year-end MAI Annual Report documenting program outcomes. Each MAI Report has two parts: (1) Web forms for standardized quantitative and qualitative information and (2) an accompanying narrative providing background information to explain the data submitted and a summary of program accomplishments, challenges, and lessons.		MAI, Part A
CARE Act Part C Grant Application	October 14, 2011	HRSA
The application requires CARE Act Part C grantees to provide information on the comprehensive continuum of outpatient HIV primary care services in the targeted area that they will provide with CARE Act and MAI funds. The application also outlines the reporting requirements and other documentation required from grantees.		Core HIV/AIDS Funding, CARE Act Part C
Federal Financial Report	Required within 90 days of the end of the budget period.	HRSA
The Federal Financial Report is an accounting of expenditures under the project that year.		Core HIV/AIDS Funding, CARE Act Part C

Administrative Requirement	Due Date, Fiscal Year 2012	Source of Grant Type of Grant
Allocation and Expenditure Reports These reports are an accounting of the allocation and expenditure of all grant funds according to the specific core medical services, support services, clinical quality management, and administration provided.	**Allocation report**: Required 60 days after the start of the budget period **Expenditure report**: Required 90 days after the end of the budget period	HRSA Core HIV/AIDS Funding, CARE Act Part C
Final Report The final report collects program-specific goals and progress on strategies; the overall impact of the project; the degree to which the grantee achieved the mission; and any barriers the grantee encountered, among other things.	Required 90 days after the end of the project period.	HRSA Core HIV/AIDS Funding, CARE Act Part C
Interim Progress Report The interim Progress report includes information on the grantee's budget, project narrative, and any additional information requested by CDC.	Due no less than 90 days after the end of the budget period	CDC Core HIV/AIDS Funding
Annual Progress Report The Annual Progress Report includes information on the progress the grantee has made in achieving the target levels for each grant objective, information on the current budget, and any other additional information CDC requests.	Due 90 days after the end of the budget period	CDC Core HIV/AIDS funding
Financial Status Report The Financial Status Report includes a final performance report and a financial status report.	Due 90 days after the end of the grant	CDC Core HIV/AIDS funding
Final Progress Report	Due 90 days after the end of the grant or no cost extension	SAMHSA MAI
Final Financial Status Report	Due 90 days after the end of the grant	SAMHSA MAI

Source: GAO analysis of HHS information.

[a]The Targeted Capacity Expansion Grant Application was due on June 13, 2011, which was in federal fiscal year 2011.

[b]The allocation report serves as a monitoring tool to track and monitor the use of grants. It identifies categories of services that are being delivered, changes in the type of services being provided over time and trends in the amount of CARE Act grants being used to deliver these services. The budget and budget justification narrative serve as monitoring tools to track and monitor the use of CARE Act grants. The implementation plan serves as a monitoring tool to verify implementation of approved medical and support services for the current grant year. The plan should include all the services and priorities reflected in the allocations report. All funded services must be included in the implementation plan. The Consolidated List of Contractors serves as a list of all subgrantees for the current grant year. The Contract Review Certification requires the grantee to certify that all subgrantees for the current grant year comply with CARE Act program requirements and federal grants requirements.

[c]The Minority AIDS Initiative Annual Report for Part A grantees was due on January 31, 2013, which is in federal fiscal year 2013.

Because of the administrative requirements associated with managing multiple HIV/AIDS grants, some grantees decided not to apply for MAI grants. In fiscal year 2011, according to information provided by HRSA, 37 percent of CARE Act Part B grantees chose not to apply for MAI grants. Some grantees that chose not to apply were states with sizeable minority populations. HRSA officials stated that several grantees reported that their reasons for not applying for MAI funds were that the small size of MAI grants did not provide enough funding to implement a program and justify the additional administrative requirements. For grantees that received several HIV/AIDS grants, including at least one MAI grant and one core HIV/AIDS grant, the average MAI grant was $391,225, while the average core HIV/AIDS grant was approximately $3,823,102. HRSA officials stated that one Part B grantee declined an MAI grant because the amount it received could not cover the cost of issuing a request for proposals for subcontractors to conduct the MAI services. A stakeholder that represents state health departments said that some states believe that due to the small amount of MAI grants they receive, it is too burdensome to justify the effort and expense to apply for and report on these grants.[32]

MAI Grantees and Stakeholder Organizations Reported a Variety of Best Practices for Community Outreach and Capacity Building

MAI grantees from our sample, as well as stakeholder organizations, reported best practices for community outreach and capacity building that at times led to improved client recruitment and improved capacity to provide care.[33]

---

[32]We found in 2009 that some Part B grantees did not apply for MAI grants because they did not think the level of funding justified the effort required to apply for and report on their use of the grants. Although MAI applications were required to be synchronized with other CARE Act grant applications in the 2009 reauthorization of the CARE Act, some Part B grantees have continued to not apply for MAI grants. GAO, *Ryan White CARE Act: Implementation of the New Minority AIDS Initiative Provisions*, GAO-09-315 (Washington, D.C.: Mar. 27, 2009).

[33]In our review of MAI services from our sample, we found that 57 out of 100 grantees reported services that we define to be best practices in their fiscal year 2011 MAI annual grantee reports. We define the term best practices to include any successes, lessons learned and/or challenges overcome that we found grantees to report regarding their MAI activities. MAI grantees generally are not required to report best practices in their annual grantee reports; therefore, our reporting of these best practices is not generalizable to the 100 grantees in our sample.

MAI Grantees and Stakeholder Organizations Reported Best Practices for Community Outreach to Improve Client Recruitment	MAI grantees from our sample of 100 grantees, as well as some of the six stakeholder organizations we interviewed, reported best practices for community outreach that included targeting specific communities, broadening outreach and education strategies, utilizing social media forums, collaborating with other organizations, and using various HIV testing strategies that at times led to increased recruitment for HIV testing and other services to communities disproportionately affected by HIV/AIDS.

- 23 grantees from our sample reported various community outreach and education services that helped some grantees improve client recruitment. For example, seven grantees offered individuals incentives (e.g., prizes, food or gift-cards) that led to increased participation in services such as testing and education. Four grantees utilized social media forums (e.g., Facebook, Twitter, online broadcasts, etc.) to conduct outreach and recruit individuals for HIV/AIDS services. Additionally, three grantees broadened their outreach and education strategies to focus on social issues that put individuals at risk for HIV/AIDS, rather than focusing specifically on HIV/AIDS, to overcome challenges with recruiting clients due to, for example, social stigmas prevalent with HIV/AIDS. One stakeholder organization we interviewed also reported tailoring outreach strategies to match the needs of targeted communities as a best practice to improve community outreach.

- 21 grantees from our sample reported strategies to target outreach and education to improve outreach to communities disproportionately affected by HIV/AIDS. For example, ten grantees conducted outreach at venues in the communities where specific minority groups or individuals at high risk for HIV/AIDS (e.g., men who have sex with men, drug users, etc.) typically congregate.

- 17 grantees from our sample reported that collaborating with other community organizations (e.g., HIV/AIDS organizations, medical providers, youth centers, juvenile detention facilities, etc.) enhanced the types of services offered to individuals. For example, six grantees established memorandums of understanding with organizations to help ensure individuals could seamlessly access services such as medical care, testing for other sexually transmitted infections and substance abuse services. Additionally, one stakeholder organization reported working with community health centers to provide culturally competent care and education to targeted minority communities.

- 15 grantees from our sample reported HIV testing strategies that they found successful in increasing HIV testing rates. For example, three grantees used rapid HIV testing methods that provided clients with immediate test results, which one grantee reported prevented potential transportation and scheduling challenges for clients to obtain test results. Three grantees also provided HIV testing services in mobile testing units, with one offering testing on evenings and weekends to make testing more convenient and accessible to clients. Additionally, one stakeholder organization reported providing HIV testing at the same event annually to establish continuity and reliability of access to HIV testing for individuals in the community.

MAI Grantees and Stakeholder Organizations Reported Capacity Building Best Practices To Improve Capacity to Provide Care

MAI grantees from our sample of 100 grantees, as well as some of the six stakeholder organizations we interviewed, reported best practices for capacity building, such as expanding infrastructure and providing training, which at times improved their capacity to provide care to communities disproportionately affected by HIV/AIDS.[34]

- Ten grantees from our sample reported activities such as training staff and expanding infrastructure that improved their ability to provide HIV/AIDS services to minority communities. For example, four grantees from our sample reported planning or conducting trainings on topics including cultural diversity which, for some grantees, improved staff's ability to provide care or conduct outreach to high-risk populations or minority communities. Two grantees also cross-trained staff to conduct different job tasks which helped to alleviate any impacts of high staff turnover. Additionally, three grantees increased their building space or service delivery areas to help expand the services they offered to clients. Two grantees also developed or enhanced their technology (e.g., databases) to track client services.

- Some stakeholder organizations that we interviewed also reported conducting evaluations and providing training to improve the capacity of organizations to provide services to minority communities. For example, some stakeholders worked with organizations such as CBOs to evaluate program needs or capacity levels in order to improve and enhance their leadership capacity and infrastructure. Additionally, some stakeholder organizations and an expert we interviewed also cited the importance of providing training to build staff skills and to build long-term capacity within organizations.

---

[34]Officials from two HHS agencies told us their MAI funds have been used to implement capacity building services to expand their ability to provide services to clients.

Conclusions

Since 1998, MAI grants have been awarded in addition to core HIV/AIDS grants in order to improve HIV-related health outcomes and reduce HIV-related health disparities for racial and ethnic minority populations. Given that the majority of individuals living with HIV/AIDS in the United States today are racial and ethnic minorities, the populations eligible for the services provided through both core HIV/AIDS grants and MAI grants are primarily minority. In most cases, MAI grants not only have the same purpose as core HIV/AIDS grants but MAI grants go to similar grantees to provide similar services. Moreover, HHS agencies and offices are required to manage separate, fragmented streams of funding that are largely intended for the same purpose.

MAI grantees face a challenge in that they are often required to complete duplicative administrative requirements for their HIV/AIDS funding. In past work, GAO has determined that federal programs are duplicative when they provide similar services to the same populations and fragmented when numerous agencies or offices provide the same services. In this case, a single department is funding the services, but it is doing so across multiple agencies and offices with multiple funding streams. Such a situation raises the possibility of inefficiencies and requires unnecessarily duplicative administrative processes of grantees that could otherwise be using their resources to provide needed services. Opportunities exist for HHS to reduce unnecessarily fragmented funding streams through its budget request and allocation process. For example, HHS can consolidate disparate MAI funding streams when making discretionary budget allocations, and it can restructure its annual budget requests to concentrate funding in core HIV/AIDS programs. HHS can also seek legislative solutions to achieve a more consolidated funding approach, for example, by amendments to the CARE Act or other law, as necessary.

Recommendations for Executive Action

In order to reduce the administrative costs associated with a fragmented MAI grant structure that diminishes the effective use of HHS's limited HIV/AIDS funding, and to enhance services to minority populations, HHS should take the following two actions:

- Consolidate disparate MAI funding streams into core HIV/AIDS funding during its budget request and allocation process, and

- Seek legislation to amend the CARE Act or other provisions of law, as necessary, to achieve a consolidated approach.

Agency Comments

We provided a copy of this report to HHS for its review and HHS provided written comments (see app. III). HHS stated that GAO's recommendations align with the National HIV/AIDS Strategy and federal program accountability goals, but also stated that any restructuring of its HIV/AIDS funding approach must ensure continued responsiveness to minorities who are disproportionately affected by HIV/AIDS. HHS welcomed an expanded discussion of strategies to more efficiently administer MAI, reduce duplicative requirements for grantees, and more effectively administer HIV/AIDS funding streams. HHS also described some of its efforts to make SMAIF more efficient, responsive, and accountable since the release of the National HIV/AIDS Strategy in July 2010.

HHS noted in its comments that it has several things to consider before it moves to restructure its HIV/AIDS core funding streams and consolidate MAI within core funding streams. HHS also noted that grantees' administrative challenges are important but aren't the only consideration in assessing the merits of funding streams and the programs they produce. HHS commented that any restructuring of core HIV/AIDS and MAI funding streams and programs must ensure that HHS maintains its responsiveness to the needs of communities and populations disproportionately impacted by the HIV/AIDS epidemic. Our recommendations that HHS take steps to consolidate disparate funding streams provide HHS with discretion in defining grant eligibility requirements or activities to address the issues HHS said it needs to consider before restructuring funding streams. Consolidation can reduce unnecessary, fragmented funding streams without compromising the issues HHS needs to consider to ensure access to services for disproportionately affected minorities.

HHS also provided technical comments, which we incorporated as appropriate.

We are sending copies of this report to the Secretary of Health and Human Services and interested congressional committees. In addition, the report is available at no charge on the GAO website at http://www.gao.gov.

If you or your staff have any questions about this report, please contact me at (202) 512-7114 or crossem@gao.gov. Contact points for our Offices of Congressional Relations and Public Affairs may be found on the last page of this report. GAO staff who made key contributions to this report are listed in appendix IV.

Marcia Crosse
Director, Health Care

The Ryan White HIV/AIDS Treatment Extension Act of 2009 requires us to report on the history of MAI program activities within each relevant Department of Health and Human Services (HHS) agency and to provide a description of activities conducted and types of grantees funded. To provide this information, we requested data from each of the HHS agencies and offices that have awarded MAI grants from 1999 through 2011 using either their own MAI program funding or transferred funding from a department-level MAI account, known as the Secretary's Minority AIDS Fund (SMAIF).[1] Three HHS agencies, the Centers for Disease Control (CDC), the Health Resources and Services Administration (HRSA), and the Substance Abuse and Mental Health Services Administration (SAMHSA), reported using their own MAI program funds to award grants to provide services in communities disproportionately affected by human immunodeficiency virus/acquired immunodeficiency syndrome (HIV/AIDS). In addition, the Office of HIV/AIDS and Infectious Disease Policy (OHAIDP), acting on behalf of the HHS Office of the Secretary, distributed SMAIF funding to HRSA, CDC, SAMHSA, and seven other HHS agencies and offices which, in turn, awarded MAI grants to provide services for communities disproportionally affected by HIV/AIDS. For HRSA, CDC and SAMSHA, we report the total funding level, by fiscal year, for their respective MAI programs as well as the total SMAIF funding they received each fiscal year. For the other seven HHS agencies, we report the total SMAIF funding they received each fiscal year.

Tables 3 and 4 show annual MAI funding from 1999 to 2011.

---

[1] In addition to grants, some agencies may have awarded MAI (including SMAIF) funding to recipients through other mechanisms such as cooperative agreements, contracts, or interagency agreements. We have treated these recipients as "grantees" for purposes of this report regardless of the funding mechanism by which they received their MAI or SMAIF funds.

Table 3: Department of Health and Human Services (HHS) Minority AIDS Initiative (MAI) Funding (in Millions of Dollars), Fiscal Years 1999-2011

Fiscal Year	Health Resources and Services Administration (HRSA)		Centers for Disease Control and Prevention (CDC)		Substance Abuse and Mental Health Services Administration (SAMHSA)	
	MAI	SMAIF[a]	MAI	SMAIF	MAI	SMAIF
1999	$22.3	$5.8	$46.9	N/A	$37.1	$12.5
2000	$73.1	$5.0	$58.7	N/A	$55.6	$12.0
2001	$109.2	$6.1	$84.4	N/A	$100.2	$11.4
2002	$123.2	$6.2	$92.9	$15.0	$110.4	$11.9
2003	$131.2	$5.6	$97.1	$13.1	$112.1	$12.0
2004	$130.3	$6.9	$97.3	$10.2	$112.0	$11.0
2005	$129.6	$8.2	$91.8	$9.7	$112.4	$11.3
2006	$128.6	$8.6	$96.1	$8.4	$111.5	$9.5
2007	$131.2	$8.6	$95.6	$7.7	$111.1	$10.2
2008	$135.1	$7.2	$94.0	$7.3	$111.7	$8.7
2009	$139.1	$5.3	$94.0	$1.8	$117.1	$9.6
2010	$146.1	$5.3	$94.0	$3.4	$116.6	$8.7
2011	$153.4	$7.7	$94.0	$10.4	$116.7	$5.9

Source: GAO analysis of Department of Health and Human Services (HHS) data.

Note: Dollar amounts are rounded to one decimal point.

[a]Secretary's Minority AIDS Initiative Fund

Table 4: Secretary's Minority AIDS Fund (SMAIF) Funding to HHS Offices (in Millions of Dollars), Fiscal Years 1999-2011

Fiscal Year	Indian Health Service	Office of Adolescent Health	Office of HIV/AIDS and Infectious Disease Policy	Office of Minority Health	Office of Population Affairs	Office on Women's Health	Regional Health Administrators
1999	$0	$0	$2.5	$5.0	$0.5	$0	$0
2000	$0.8	$0	$3.0	$6.5	$0.6	$0.5	$0
2001	$1.1	$0	$3.4	$7.8	$3.0	$0.5	$0
2002	$1.5	$0	$3.2	$7.9	$3.0	$0.6	$0
2003	$1.5	$0	$3.2	$7.9	$3.0	$0.6	$0
2004	$1.5	$0	$3.2	$7.7	$6.0	$1.6	$0
2005	$2.1	$0	$3.0	$7.7	$6.0	$3.1	$0
2006	$2.0	$0	$6.0	$7.0	$6.1	$3.0	$0
2007	$1.9	$0	$4.3	$6.8	$6.0	$4.0	$0
2008	$2.3	$0	$2.2	$8.8	$7.1	$4.0	$1.3
2009	$3.2	$0	$3.3	$8.9	$8.1	$6.1	$1.8
2010	$4.4	$0	$3.7	$8.9	$7.9	$7.0	$1.7
2011	$4.2	$0.2	$3.4	$5.5	$7.2	$3.4	$2.0

Source: GAO analysis of Department of Health and Human Services (HHS) data.

Note: The National Institutes of Health is not listed in the chart above because it only received funding from the Secretary's Minority AIDS Initiative Fund in fiscal years 1999 and 2000. It received $2.7 million in fiscal year 1999 and $1.2 million in fiscal year 2000. Dollar amounts are rounded to one decimal point.

HRSA

HRSA's MAI program was codified into law pursuant to the 2006 reauthorization of the Ryan White Comprehensive AIDS Resources Emergency Act of 1990 (CARE Act).[2] To be eligible for MAI grants under the CARE Act, grantees must also have received grants under other provisions of the CARE Act. HRSA reserves amounts from its annual CARE Act appropriation for making supplemental MAI grants. There are five primary sections of the CARE Act under which HRSA awards grants, including MAI grants—Parts A, B, C, D and F. According to HRSA,

- Part A MAI provides for grants to selected metropolitan areas—known as eligible metropolitan areas and transitional grant areas—that have

[2]See Ryan White HIV/AIDS Treatment Modernization Act of 2006, Pub. L. No. 109-415, § 603, 120 Stat. 2767, 2818 (codified at 42 U.S.C. § 300ff-121).

been disproportionately affected by the HIV/AIDS epidemic.[3] Part A MAI grantees provide outpatient medical care, mental health and oral health services, local pharmacy assistance, substance abuse treatment, outreach, case management, early intervention services, treatment adherence, and health education/risk reduction.

- Part B MAI provides for grants to states and territories. Part B grantees provide targeted outreach and educational activities to increase minority participation in the AIDS Drug Assistance Program.

- Part C MAI provides for grants to community health centers, health departments, hospitals, medical centers and community-based organizations (CBOs). Part C MAI grantees provide outpatient early invention services including: primary medical care, oral health care, mental health screening and treatment, substance abuse screening and treatment, adherence counseling, nutritional services, and specialty care.

- Part D MAI provides for grants to state health departments, hospitals or university based clinics, and other CBOs. Part D MAI grantees provide family centered outpatient primary medical care, oral health care, mental health screening and treatment, substance abuse, screening and treatment, adherence counseling, nutritional services, specialty care, pediatric care, women's health, and access to clinical trials.

- Part D Youth MAI provides grants to hospitals, universities and other CBOs. Part D Youth grantees identify HIV infected youth who are not in care; enroll them in medical and supportive care; and retain them in care. They also provide family centered outpatient primary medical care, oral health care, mental health screening and treatment, substance abuse screening and treatment, adherence counseling, nutritional services, specialty care, and access to clinical trials.

- Part F provides for grants to hospitals and universities. Part F MAI grantees provide technical assistance, training, and education to other MAI grantees.

---

[3]Eligible metropolitan areas are areas that have a population of 50,000 persons or more and had a cumulative total of more than 2,000 new AIDS cases during the most recent 5-year period. Transitional grant areas are areas that have a population of 50,000 persons or more and had a cumulative total of 1,000 to 1,999 new AIDS cases during the most recent 5-year period.

HRSA reported that it also received SMAIF funding which it used for grants for outreach to minority populations and training to HIV providers, contracts promoting linkages to care for HIV/AIDS clients, and cooperative agreements to support networks of HIV care by enhancing primary medical care. HRSA's SMAIF funding was also used in connection with interagency agreements with CDC and its HIV/AIDS Bureau. (See HRSA funding amounts and number of organizations funded in table 5.)

Table 5: Health Resources and Services Administration (HRSA) Minority AIDS Initiative Funding (in Millions of Dollars) and Number of Grantees, by Part, Fiscal Years 2007-2011

Ryan White Part	2007		2008		2009		2010		2011	
	Funding	Number of Grantees	Funding	Number of Grantees	Funding	Number of Grantees	Funding	Number of Grantees	Funding	Number of Grantees
Part A	$43.8	56	$45.4	56	$47.1	56	$46.7	56	$49.1	52
Part B	$7.0	30	$7.3	26	$7.5	26	$8.8	36	$9.2	36
Part C	$53.4	206	$55.4	208	$57.4	204	$61.3	203	$64.4	212
Part D	$17.1	57	$17.1	55	$17.2	58	$18.9	58	$20.0	61
Part D Youth	$1.4	10	$1.4	10	$1.4	10	$1.5	10	$1.5	10
Part F	$8.5	15	$8.5	15	$8.5	15	$8.8	15	$9.2	16
SMAIF[a]	$8.6	24	$7.2	20	$5.3	26	$5.3	19	$7.7	33

Source: GAO analysis of HRSA and Office of HIV/AIDS and Infectious Disease Policy data.

Note: Dollar amounts are rounded to one decimal point.

[a]Secretary's Minority AIDS Initiative Fund.

CDC

In fiscal year 2007-2011 CDC reported that it awarded MAI funding through cooperative agreements, contracts, interagency agreements, and grants. Organizations that are awarded MAI funds by CDC include business and commercial vendors, colleges and universities, CBOs, federal agencies, hospitals, health departments, and national or regional organizations. These organizations used MAI awards to provide capacity building, evaluation, HIV prevention, demonstration projects, and research activities to individuals disproportionately affected by HIV/AIDS.

CDC reported that it awarded SMAIF funding through contracts, cooperative agreements and interagency agreements to a federal agency and a national/regional organization, health departments, universities, business/commercial vendors, and CBOs for capacity building, evaluation, HIV prevention, surveillance, demonstration projects, and research efforts. (See CDC funding amounts and number of organizations funded in table 6.)

Table 6: Centers for Disease Control and Prevention (CDC) Minority AIDS Initiative (MAI) Funding (in Millions of Dollars) and Number of Grantees, Fiscal Years 2007-2011

Fiscal Year	MAI	Number of Grantees	SMAIF[a]	Number of Grantees
2007	$95.6	239	$7.7	36
2008	$94.0	241	$7.3	27
2009	$94.0	252	$1.8	5
2010	$94.0	218	$3.4	29
2011	$94.0	217	$10.4	60

Source: GAO analysis of CDC and Office of HIV/A DS and Infectious Disease Policy data.

Note: Dollar amounts are rounded to one decimal point.

[a]Secretary's Minority AIDS Initiative Fund.

SAMHSA

SAMHSA reported that they award MAI grants through three Centers: the Center for Mental Health Services, the Center for Substance Abuse Prevention, and the Center for Substance Abuse Treatment.

- The Center for Mental Health Services reported that in fiscal years 2007-2010 it awarded cooperative agreements to domestic public and private nonprofit entities. These cooperative agreements are intended to enhance and expand the provision of effective, culturally competent HIV/AIDS-related mental health services in minority communities for persons living with HIV/AIDS and having a mental health need. In fiscal year 2011, SAMHSA awarded funds to city and state health departments in 11 cities, specifically among recipients of the CDC's Enhanced Comprehensive HIV Prevention Planning and Implementation for Metropolitan Statistical Areas Most Affected by HIV/AIDS grant program. According to agency documentation, these entities intended to ensure that individuals that are either at high risk for or have a mental or substance use disorder, and who are most at risk for or are living with HIV/AIDS, had access to and received appropriate behavioral health services (including prevention and treatment), HIV/AIDS care, and medical treatment in integrated behavioral health and primary care settings. Under this project, activities were also targeted to integrate behavioral health and primary care networks for HIV and medical treatment in minority communities.

- The Center for Substance Abuse Treatment reported that in fiscal years 2007-2010 it awarded grants to CBOs, faith-based organizations, national organizations, colleges and universities, clinics and hospitals, research institutions, state and local government agencies, and tribal entities to enhance and expand substance abuse treatment and/or outreach and pretreatment services in conjunction with HIV/AIDS services in African-American, Latino/Hispanic, and/or other racial or ethnic communities highly affected by substance abuse and HIV/AIDS. According to agency documentation, the Center also awarded SMAIF grants to cohorts of organizations to expand the capacity for providers to deliver rapid HIV testing, counseling and referrals to care for fiscal year 2011.

- The Center for Substance Abuse Prevention reported that in fiscal years 2007-2011 it awarded cooperative agreements to CBOs targeting at risk minority populations as well as colleges and universities to provide a variety of activities including substance abuse prevention services, HIV testing and outreach services; pre-post counseling, reentry programs hepatitis education, and technical assistance. Additionally, in this same timeframe contracts were awarded for the review of grants, evaluation activity, technical assistance to MAI grantees such as faith-based and community organizations and the organization of grantee meetings. The Center also awarded contracts to for-profit organizations and tribal organizations with SMAIF funding during fiscal years 2007-2011. For example, according to agency documentation, these organizations provided training and technical assistance to coordinate substance abuse education, HIV outreach and awareness, as well as testing on college campuses and universities. (See SAMHSA funding and number of grantees funded in Table 7.)

Table 7: Substance Abuse and Mental Health Services Administration (SAMHSA) Minority AIDS Initiative (MAI) Funding (in Millions of Dollars) and Number of Grantees, Fiscal Years 2007-2011

Fiscal Year	MAI	Number of Grantees	SMAIF[a]	Number of Grantees[b]
2007	$111.1	287	$10.2	115
2008	$111.7	276	$8.7	133
2009	$117.1	295	$9.6	148
2010	$116.6	275	$8.7	142
2011	$116.7	269	$5.9	139

Source: GAO analysis of SAMHSA and Office of HIV/AIDS and Infectious Disease Policy data.

Note: Dollar amounts are rounded to one decimal point.

[a]Secretary's Minority AIDS Initiative Fund.

[b]Some of SAMHSA's grants were funded with both MAI and SMAIF funds.

Indian Health Service (IHS)

IHS reported that it awarded SMAIF funding through grants, cooperative agreements, contracts and interagency agreements in fiscal years 2007 through 2011. Specifically, the agency reported that Urban Indian Health programs received grants to provide HIV screening services and IHS established interagency agreements with federal sites for capacity building and access to care services. Additionally, contractors provided capacity building services, online HIV training for clinicians, and educational videos. Cooperative agreements, grants, and interagency agreements were made to increase HIV screening services. Lastly, grants were used to provide effective behavioral interventions for tribal communities. (See IHS MAI funding and number of grantees funded in table 8.)

Table 8: Indian Health Service (IHS) Secretary's Minority AIDS Initiative Funding (in Millions of Dollars) and Number of Grantees, Fiscal Years 2007-2011

Fiscal Year	SMAIF[a]	Number of Grantees
2007	$1.9	11
2008	$2.3	19
2009	$3.2	42
2010	$4.4	31
2011	$4.2	46

Source: GAO analysis of Office of HIV/AIDS and Infectious Disease Policy and IHS data.

Note: Dollar amounts are rounded to one decimal point.

[a]Secretary's Minority AIDS Initiative Fund.

Office of Adolescent Health (OAH)

OAH reported that it received $200,000 in SMAIF funding in fiscal year 2011 that it used for a cooperative agreement with a university to provide management of a resource center website and technical assistance. OAH did not receive SMAIF funds prior to fiscal year 2011.

OHAIDP

OHAIDP reported that it used its SMAIF funding to award contracts to national technology and health communications firms and consultants to provide technical assistance, education, and outreach via AIDS.gov during fiscal years 2007-2011. (See OHAIDP funding amounts and number of organizations funded in table 9.) Additionally, CBOs and faith-based organizations, health departments, universities and colleges, and training centers were awarded contracts by OHAIDP. These entities provided outreach, education, technical assistance, HIV testing, and capacity building for the Minority Serving Institutions HIV/AIDS Prevention Demonstration Initiative. OHAIDP officials also reported that SMAIF funds were used for the National HIV testing mobilization campaign, and to coordinate for the National HIV/AIDS Strategy during this timeframe.

Table 9: Office of HIV/AIDS and Infectious Disease Policy (OHAIDP) Secretary's Minority AIDS Initiative Funding (in Millions of Dollars) and Number of Grantees, Fiscal Years 2007-2011

Fiscal Year	SMAIF[a]	Number of Grantees
2007	$4.3	6
2008	$2.2	7
2009	$3.3	11
2010	$3.7	13
2011	$3.4	12

Source: GAO analysis of OHAIDP data.

Note: Dollar amounts are rounded to one decimal point.

[a]Secretary's Minority AIDS Initiative Fund.

HHS Office of Minority Health (OMH)

OMH reported that it used its SMAIF funding to award grants and cooperative agreements to CBOs and national organizations during fiscal years 2007 through 2011. (See OMH funding amounts and number of organizations funded in table 10.) Specifically, these funding mechanisms provided capacity building, technical assistance, health promotion and education, access to testing and care, counseling, peer education, and links to social and support services.

Table 10: Office of Minority Health (OMH) Secretary's Minority AIDS Initiative Funding (in Millions of Dollars) and Number of Grantees, Fiscal Years 2007-2011

Fiscal Year	SMAIF[a]	Number of Grantees
2007	$6.8	24
2008	$8.8	42
2009	$8.9	51
2010	$8.9	43
2011	$5.5	34

Source: GAO analysis of Office of HIV/AIDS and Infectious Disease Policy and OMH data.

Note: Dollar amounts are rounded to one decimal point.

[a]Secretary's Minority AIDS Initiative Fund.

Office of Population Affairs (OPA)

OPA reported that it used its SMAIF funding to award grants to health departments, community health centers, Planned Parenthood, as well as other organizations including non-profits, universities, hospitals, faith-based organizations, tribal health centers, and free-standing family planning organizations during fiscal years 2007 through 2011. (See OPA funding amounts and number of organizations funded in table 11.) Specifically, these grants provided for expanded HIV testing, prevention education, and referrals to care.

Table 11: Office of Population Affairs (OPA) Secretary's Minority AIDS Initiative Funding (in Millions of Dollars) and Number of Grantees, Fiscal Years 2007-2011

Fiscal Year	SMAIF[a]	Number of Grantees
2007	$6.0	47
2008	$7.1	50
2009	$8.1	51
2010	$7.9	54
2011	$7.2	54

Source: GAO analysis of Office of HIV/AIDS and Infectious Disease Policy and OPA data.

Note: Dollar amounts are rounded to one decimal point.

[a]Secretary's Minority AIDS Initiative Fund.

Office on Women's Health (OWH)

OWH reported that it used its SMAIF funding in fiscal years 2007-2011 to award grants for HIV prevention and education services for women, including adolescents and youths at risk of HIV/AIDS. OWH reported that SMAIF funds were used for contracts and cooperative agreements to provide services to women living in the United States Virgin Islands,

Puerto Rico, and Native American women, as well as women sexually involved with an incarcerated or recently released partner. (See OWH funding and number of grantees funded in table 12.) Additionally, OWH awarded grants for outreach and education services and events including the National HIV/AIDS Awareness Day and the Young Women's Mobilization project.

Table 12: Office on Women's Health (OWH) Secretary's Minority AIDS Initiative Funding (in Millions of Dollars) and Number of Grantees, Fiscal Years 2007-2011

Fiscal Year	SMAIF[a]	Number of Grantees
2007	$4.0	36
2008	$4.0	37
2009	$6.1	50
2010	$7.0	43
2011	$3.4	30

Source: GAO analysis of Office of HIV/AIDS and Infectious Disease Policy and OWH data.

Note: Dollar amounts are rounded to one decimal point.

[a]Secretary's Minority AIDS Initiative Fund.

Regional Health Administrators (RHA)

RHA reported that it used its SMAIF funding to contract with a for-profit, publicly owned, and traded company to provide capacity building services in fiscal years 2008-2011. (See RHA funding and number of grantees funded in table 13.)

Table 13: Regional Health Administrators (RHA) Secretary's Minority AIDS Initiative Funding (in Millions of Dollars) and Number of Grantees, Fiscal Years 2007-2011

Fiscal Year	SMAIF[a]	Number of Grantees
2007	$0	0
2008	$1.3	1
2009	$1.8	1
2010	$1.7	1
2011	$2.0	1

Source: GAO analysis of Office of HIV/AIDS and Infectious Disease Policy and RHA data.

Note: Dollar amounts are rounded to one decimal point.

[a]Secretary's Minority AIDS Initiative Fund.

Appendix II: Methodology for Review of Minority AIDS Initiative (MAI) Services from Sample of MAI Annual Grantee Reports

To identify the types of services provided by grantees under MAI, we selected a generalizable sample from 100 fiscal year 2011 grantees in order to review their MAI annual grantee reports. To select our sample, we created a list of all MAI grantees from the ten Department of Health and Human Services (HHS) agencies and offices that awarded MAI grants in fiscal year 2011.[1] We selected a generalizable sample of 100 grantees that were approximately proportional to MAI funding amounts for the respective agencies and offices. We then requested fiscal year 2011 MAI annual grantee reports for the 100 grantees from these agencies and offices and uploaded the reports into NVivo.[2] This sample is generalizable to the whole population of MAI grantees. The sample was selected within agency strata, with strata sample sizes defined to ensure that the distribution of grantee spending for each agency was approximately proportional to its distribution in the population of grantees. We calculated sampling weights that reflected this design, which allowed us to appropriately combine data across the agency strata and make estimates that generalized to the whole population of MAI grantees.

We used NVivo to conduct a review of MAI services using the MAI annual grantee reports we obtained from the generalizable sample of 100 MAI grantees we selected.[3,4] In order to identify the types of MAI services, we categorized MAI services into six categories based on an initial review of the reports: (1) administrative; (2) medical services; (3) client assistance; (4) community outreach/education; (5) training; and (6) testing. We

---

[1]We identified a total of 1067 organizations awarded MAI grants by the ten HHS agencies and offices in fiscal year 2011. In addition to grants, some agencies may have awarded MAI funding to recipients through other mechanisms such as cooperative agreements, contracts, or interagency agreements. We have treated these recipients as "grantees" for purposes of this report regardless of the funding mechanism by which they received their funds. Fiscal year 2011 was the most recent year that grantee data was available for most HHS agencies and offices.

[2]We obtained fiscal year 2010 MAI annual grantee reports for some grantees who had not yet submitted their fiscal year 2011 reports. We reviewed all grantee reports in our sample for accuracy and to ensure they contained information on MAI services.

[3]NVivo is a qualitative data analysis software system that allows organization and analysis of information from a variety of sources including complex nonnumeric or unstructured data.

[4]MAI grantees submit annual grantee reports to the agency that awarded their MAI grants that typically include information on the types of services they provide with their MAI grants. Grantees that receive more than one MAI grant often have to submit a separate report to each agency from which they receive funds.

created an additional category to identify best practices reported by grantees to inform our second objective on best practices for community outreach and capacity building of community-based organizations serving communities that are disproportionately affected by human immunodeficiency virus/acquired immunodeficiency syndrome (HIV/AIDS). We defined the term best practices to include any successes, lessons learned, or challenges overcome by grantees regarding their MAI activities. We also created sub-categories for medical services and best practices in order to obtain more detailed information on these categories (see table 14 for the definitions of MAI categories and sub-categories).

Table 14: Categories of Services and Best Practices Identified in MAI Annual Grantee Reports

Category	Definition
Administrative	Grantee performs activities to help maintain its ability to conduct MAI activities, daily procedures and operation including assisting providers or other organizations in planning or implementing MAI activities, providing technical assistance, collaborating with organizations, etc.
Medical Services	Grantee provides or assists in providing direct medical services to clients, including dental, substance abuse, mental health, etc.
	Sub-categories
	• HIV Primary and Outpatient Care: grantee provides primary care to clients in an inpatient or outpatient setting.
	• Substance Abuse Treatment/Counseling: grantee provides substance abuse treatment or care to clients in an inpatient or outpatient setting.
	• Mental Health Treatment/Counseling: grantee provides mental health treatment or counseling to clients in an inpatient or outpatient setting.
	• Screening/Testing for other sexually transmitted infections: grantee screens or tests clients for sexually transmitted diseases besides HIV.
	• Administrative/Collaboration: grantee assists or collaborates with providers who provide direct medical services.
Client Assistance	Grantee provides or assists providers in facilitating, referring or supporting client's care coordination, case management, counseling, as well as assisting clients with obtaining social services.
Community Outreach/ Education	Grantee provides or assists in providing outreach and education services to clients and individuals with HIV/AIDS through social media, marketing, community events, training, etc.
Training	Grantee provides or receives training for grantee staff, providers, other organizations, etc.
Testing	Grantee directly provides or assists providers with clients testing services for HIV/AIDS, or other related illnesses.
Best Practices	Grantee cites any best practices, lessons learned and/or challenges overcome related to their MAI activities.

Category	Definition
	Sub-categories
	• Collaboration: grantee cites collaborating with other organizations that aided its ability to provide services to clients.
	• Targeted Community Outreach/Education: grantee cites activities that are specifically targeted to improve outreach to communities disproportionately affected by HIV/AIDS.
	• Community Outreach/Education: grantee cites activities to improve outreach and marketing to clients.
	• Client Assistance: grantee cites activities to help improve or facilitate linking clients to care, social support or medical services.
	• Testing: grantee cites activities to encourage clients to get tested for HIV/AIDS/other sexually transmitted infections.
	• Medical Services: grantee cites activities to improve their ability to provide or facilitate medical care for their clients.
	• Capacity Building: grantee cites activities to improve their infrastructure and expand their ability to provide services to clients.
	• Administrative: grantee cites activities to help maintain its ability to conduct MAI activities, daily procedures and operation.

Source: GAO.

We conducted a review of MAI services from the sample of 100 MAI annual grantee reports in which three members of the team independently coded a selection of reports to identify MAI services. We reviewed each other's coding to ensure its accuracy and resolved any disagreements or inconsistencies in coding through a discussion between team members to ensure mutual agreement that the services identified in the annual grantee reports were consistent with the categories of services listed in Table 14 above.

We identified the services provided in the 100 MAI annual grantee reports through several rounds of NVivo coding and review. We then analyzed our coding results in order to identify the types and frequency of MAI services conducted by MAI grantees in our sample. We analyzed and compared the MAI services identified in the six categories by grant amount, HHS agency and office (e.g., the Health Resources and Services Administration, Centers for Disease Control and Prevention, etc.), source of grant (e.g., agency MAI allocation or funding from the Secretary's MAI Fund) and organization type (e.g., community-based organization, city, etc). We also analyzed the output to identify best practices reported by grantees that were associated with providing MAI services and/or in serving communities disproportionally affected by HIV/AIDS. However, because MAI grantees generally were not required to discuss best practices in their annual grantee reports, we could not estimate the proportion of grantees identifying such practices and, as a result, our estimates are not generalizeable for this purpose.

Estimates of the services provided and population served from this sample are generalizable to the population of MAI grantees. We summarize the statistical precision of our estimates using a 95 percent confidence interval, which is the interval that would contain the population value in 95 percent of the samples we could have drawn. Since the size of the confidence intervals varies widely across the estimates, we specify these intervals where we refer to the estimates.

Appendix III: Comments from the Department of Health and Human Services

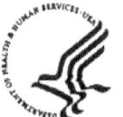

DEPARTMENT OF HEALTH & HUMAN SERVICES   OFFICE OF THE SECRETARY

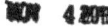

Assistant Secretary for Legislation
Washington, DC 20201

JUN 4 2013

Marcia Crosse
Director, Health Care
U.S. Government Accountability Office
441 G Street NW
Washington, DC 20548

Dear Ms. Crosse:

Attached are comments on the U.S. Government Accountability Office's (GAO) report entitled, "Minority Aids Initiative: Consolidation of Fragmented HIV/AIDS Funding Could Reduce Administrative Challenges" (GAO-14-84).

The Department appreciates the opportunity to review this report prior to publication.

Sincerely,

Jim R. Esquea
Assistant Secretary for Legislation

Attachment

<u>**GENERAL COMMENTS OF THE DEPARTMENT OF HEALTH AND HUMAN
SERVICES (HHS) ON THE GOVERNMENT ACCOUNTABILITY OFFICE'S (GAO)
DRAFT REPORT ENTITLED, "MINORITY AIDS INITIATIVE (MAI):
CONSOLIDATION OF FRAGMENTED FUNDING COULD REDUCE
ADMINISTRATIVE CHALLENGES" (GAO-14-84)**</u>

The Department appreciates the opportunity to review and comment on this draft report.

HHS welcomes an expanded discussion on strategies to improve the administrative efficiencies
of the Minority AIDS Initiative (MAI) including the Secretary's Minority AIDS Initiative Fund
(SMAIF); reduce duplicative application, data collection and reporting requirements and burdens
on grantees; reduce programmatic redundancy; and otherwise improve effective administration
of HHS HIV/AIDS funding streams, both "core" and MAI. To address these administrative
challenges, the GAO Report recommends that: (1) HHS "consolidate disparate MAI funding
streams into core funding during its budget request and allocation process; and (2) seek
legislation to amend the CARE Act or other provisions of law, as necessary to achieve a
consolidated approach." These administrative improvements appear to be in alignment with the
National HIV/AIDS Strategy and more overarching federal program accountability
goals. However, before we move to restructure our HIV/AIDS core funding streams and
consolidate the MAI within core funding streams, HHS would like to provide the following
considerations.

Any proposed restructuring of HIV/AIDS funding involving the elimination or consolidation of
MAI, should take into account the original impetus and intent of the MAI including the
acknowledgement that it was dissatisfaction with the use of "core HIV/AIDS funding" that
prompted community leaders, members of Congress, and ultimately President Clinton to
advocate for this racially and ethnically targeted funding. The original goals of the MAI are to
improve HIV-related health outcomes and improve HIV-related health disparities among racial
and ethnic minorities by increasing capacity of indigenous minority community based
organizations to more effectively serve their communities. Innovative and successful strategies
targeted at the highest risk and hardest to serve populations were encouraged. The extent to
which these goals remain viable and achievable in the absence of MAI funding should be
considered.

Related to the point above, administrative challenges are important but they aren't the only
consideration in assessing the merits of funding streams and the programs they produce. Any
restructuring of the core and MAI HIV/AIDS funding streams must ensure that HHS continues to
be responsive to the HIV/AIDS needs of communities and populations disproportionately
impacted by this epidemic. While all Americans should benefit from the broader public health
programs, services, campaigns and activities that anchor "core HIV/AIDS funding," we must
keep in mind that we don't have a generalized epidemic in the US. Certain racial and ethnic
minority populations and specific sexual minority populations are at greater risk and have been
disproportionately impacted. We should strive to be comprehensive and strategic in our reforms
not simply efficient. The assessment of the administrative challenges says nothing about how
responsive the programs are to the epidemic nor if the services or activities are appropriately
prioritized, targeted and accountable.

It should be noted that with the exception of CDC, HRSA and SAMHSA, the SMAIF is the
primary or sole source of HIV funding for IHS and the 6 OASH offices (OMH, OWH, OHAIDP,

1

**GENERAL COMMENTS OF THE DEPARTMENT OF HEALTH AND HUMAN
SERVICES (HHS) ON THE GOVERNMENT ACCOUNTABILITY OFFICE'S (GAO)
DRAFT REPORT ENTITLED, "MINORITY AIDS INITIATIVE (MAI):
CONSOLIDATION OF FRAGMENTED FUNDING COULD REDUCE
ADMINISTRATIVE CHALLENGES" (GAO-14-84)**

OAH, OPA, & RHA). Consolidation to core HIV/AIDS funding will likely reduce the number
of agencies or offices providing HIV/AIDS programming. The potential repercussions of this
change on the Indian Health Service programming, our regional outreach and education efforts,
the integration of HIV testing in our family planning clinics, and other MAI-funded
programming must be considered.

To illustrate the MAI fragmentation within a jurisdiction, the Report examines the city of
Chicago and suggests that other cities like Philadelphia, San Francisco, Los Angeles and New
York confront a similar array of fragmented grants with multiple administrative
requirements. The suggestion is that the grants all provide the same basic HIV/AIDS prevention
and treatment services. We caution against assuming redundancy without a more comprehensive
and nuanced review of what services are actually being provided, for whom, where and
how. Chicago, like the other four cities is a geographically large, dense and diverse city. The
racial, ethnic, cultural, and linguistic mix of residents needing HIV/AIDS programs and services
could not be met with a one-size fits all approach. We must be vigilant to ensure that our efforts
to improve administrative efficiency don't sacrifice a responsive, targeted approach.

Since the release of the NHAS in July 2010, several changes have been made in the
administration of the SMAIF that have made the use of these funds more efficient, responsive
and accountable. Over the last few years, OHAIDP has completed a restructuring on the
administrative guidance and programmatic use of the SMAIF. These improvements include the
development of a funding opportunity announcement (FOA) for use by the several agencies and
offices that compete for SMAIF resources for their proposed projects. In addition to delineating
priority project areas and targeted populations, the FOA outlines specific conditions of award
that encourage cross-agency collaboration and require the integration of core indicators, data
streamlining, and a reduction in reporting requirements as now expected with all HIV/AIDS
programming. In addition, the use of larger scale, cross-agency demonstration initiatives such as
the 12 Cities Demo, Care and Prevention of HIV in the US (CAPUS), and the soon to be released
HIV Care Continuum Demo are all SMAIF-funded initiatives that specifically address concerns
over multiple application, data collection and reporting requirements. Finally, due to a
reassessment of their role in direct program and service delivery, OASH offices, including OMH,
OWH and OHAIDP, have experienced a reduction in the number of HIV/AIDS projects funded
over the last five years from the SMAIF.

2

Appendix IV: GAO Contact and Staff Acknowledgments

GAO Contact	Marcia Crosse, (202) 512-7114 or crossem@gao.gov
Acknowledgments	In addition to the contact named above, key contributors to this report were Tom Conahan, Assistant Director; Romonda McKinney Bumpus; Cathleen Hamann; Seta Hovagimian; Jessica Morris; Steven Putansu; Jeff Tessin; and Jennifer Whitworth.

www.ingramcontent.com/pod-product-compliance
Lightning Source LLC
Chambersburg PA
CBHW080615290526
45790CB00007B/2791